Barbers, Cars, and Cigars

Activity Programming for Older Men

by

Nancy Dezan

Coypright 1992 Nancy Dezan

First printing 1992 · Second printing 1993
Third printing 1994 · Fourth printing 1995
Fifth printing 1996 · Sixth printing 1997
Seventh printing 1999

All rights reserved. No part of this book may reproduced without permission of the publisher.

For additional copies or a free catalog, write to the publisher.

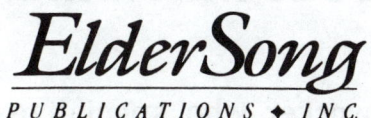

P.O. Box 74
Mt. Airy, Maryland 21771

Cover illustration by Linda Gibbon

Printed in the U.S.A.

ISBN 1-879633-12-4

Dedication

This book is dedicated to my loving husband John, and to the members of the Friends Club of Washington, D.C., who inspired this writing.

About the Author

Nancy Dezan is a social worker who specializes in assisting families and individuals with Alzheimer's disease. Her experience includes several years of directing activities in nursing homes and adult day care programs. From 1982-1989, Nancy was Executive Director of the Bethesda Fellowship House, an adult day care program in Bethesda, Maryland, which primarily serves individuals with dementia. Currently, she is a private consultant and conducts a weekly group with men in the early stages of Alzheimer's disease.

Contents

Introduction 1

Chapter 1 - Meaningful Experiences 3

Chapter 2 - Intergenerational Programming 5

Chapter 3 - Man and His Newspaper 9

Chapter 4 - Reminiscing 14

    Men's Clothing and Accessories 16

    World War II 18

    The Great Depression 20

    Movies and Entertainment 22

    Radio 24

    Automobiles 26

    Planes and Trains 28

    Occupations 30

Chapter 5 - Music 32

Chapter 6 - Men and Food 34

Chapter 7 - Sports 37

Chapter 8 - Active Games 43

Chapter 9 - Women Men Have Loved 46

One Last Thought - Don't Forget Father's Day! 49

Resource List 50

Introduction

Why write a book of activities just for men? Over the years, I have become increasingly convinced that men are often shortchanged when it comes to activity programming in long-term care. The majority of participants in nursing homes, adult day care centers, and even senior centers are women. These women often adapt to social situations more readily. They are frequently more verbal, allowing them to dominate discussion groups and to direct conversation to topics that interest them. And while there are many excellent male activity coordinators, most of the individuals who plan and implement social functions for the elderly are female. No wonder many men feel isolated in long-term care facilities and are reluctant to join the group!

Most capable, hard-working activity coordinators recognize that men may have different interests than women and need their own type of programming. In discussion groups, activity coordinators may introduce "men's" topics, such as "automobiles," "sports," and "experiences in World War II," but men's needs go beyond these efforts. This book is designed to assist the group leader in developing men's groups and, further, in understanding and meeting the needs of the men in these groups.

I believe men approach life in an entirely different fashion than women. When discussing sports, for example, I've observed that men talk about statistics and challenging play. While women also enjoy the game, they might focus on player relationships or even style of uniform. In a mixed group, a sports discussion might only continue for a short period of time but last an hour in an all male gathering.

Group leaders should encourage the men to direct the activity as much as they are able. During a recent discussion on automobiles, I displayed several pictures of old cars for my men's group. While I was focusing on style, color, and the use of a rumble seat, the men spent nearly an hour discussing differences in fenders and grillwork from one year to the next. Later they discussed horsepower and gas mileage. These men, all diagnosed with Alzheimer's disease, recalled these very specific details because they were important to them. When the group leader focuses on what is important to the men, he or she serves to build self-esteem and to create an atmosphere of enjoyment among group members.

In nearly all cases, men who are currently senior citizens grew up in an age where they were expected to be the "breadwinners." Wives often stayed home to raise the family while the men controlled the finances. Men *expect* to be in control—of themselves, their families, their jobs, and their lives. As one ages, one slowly loses control of many things. If an impairment such as dementia is added, the loss becomes devastating. Not only does he lose identity, independence, and freedom, he also loses his most important asset—the ability to reason and think. As a result, he may feel insecure, threatened, inferior, frightened, depressed, and out of control. He may continually ask, "Where is my job? I need to go to work!" He needs to be needed, in large part, because he has learned to define himself through his work.

One of the most difficult jobs an activity coordinator faces is that of helping a participant feel worthwhile and needed. Through this book I hope to provide ideas for meaningful, adult activity that will help the men in your facility find friendship, expand their skills, help others, and focus on something other than their own disabilities.

General Suggestions for Forming a Men's Group

1. Give your group a catchy title. Refer to it as a club or something familiar to the men in your facility.

2. The ideal group is small, 12-15 men. It is best if the same men attend each gathering so that a bond can be formed between group members.

3. If appropriate, send invitations for the men to join the group or personally invite them to the initial gathering.

4. Explore the men's interests, past work history, and family life. Encourage group members to share common interests. Provide name tags so that they can refer to each other by name.

5. Meet in the same room or area for each gathering. If many of the men were businessmen, you may choose to have the initial part of each gathering around a table as if it were a business meeting of sorts. This time can be used to discuss future plans and activities.

6. Take a personal interest in the men. If one has become ill, have the club members send a card. Recognize club member's birthdays and special occasions. Encourage friendship between the members.

The following chapters present activities and topics that are of special interest to men. Material is presented particularly for the activity coordinator who may have had little exposure to such themes. Be aware that not all men are necessarily interested in these subjects and that these selected subjects are certainly not the only areas of interest for men. The key is to know your group and their interests.

The suggested programs can be effective with both alert and cognitively-impaired older adults. In nearly every chapter, "suggested props" are listed to help encourage memories and enliven the program. These pictures and items from the past are essential if conducting a program with individuals diagnosed with dementia. Props serve to wake up the senses and invigorate memories. Helpful resources are mentioned throughout the book, with a complete resource list in the back. All of the book resources mentioned have been found in community libraries.

Chapter 1

Meaningful Experiences

Some men look forward to retirement. For others, it is the beginning of the end. Having once been the hard-working family breadwinner, it is often difficult for men (and women) to spend long hours participating in leisure activity. And this becomes even more difficult when compounded with dementia or a physical disability.

Finding meaningful experiences for men can be challenging. Most individuals, even those who are cognitively-impaired, know when they have been given "busy" work. Others may be insulted with the type of job provided.

Recently, when working with a group of men (all in the early stages of Alzheimer's disease), I realized that their meeting room desperately needed painting. What a wonderful idea! Have the men (with assistance) paint their own room! Wrong. When I proposed the idea, several of the men suggested we hire a painter. These had all been professional men who had never needed to paint their own homes. They had always hired someone else and were rather insulted at my suggestion. For them, this would not be a meaningful experience. In the final analysis, I actually did find two men who were the "handyman" type and who thoroughly enjoyed the task. Several volunteers were required to help them out but, for these two, painting the room was an extremely meaningful experience. They are reminded of their accomplishment every time they enter the meeting room.

Suggestions for Meaningful Experiences

Start a Service Project

Contact a local "soup kitchen" or similar facility designed to feed homeless individuals and ask what you can do to help. Our men's group makes 100 cheese sandwiches each week for a local shelter. The shelter provides the bread and plastic sandwich bags, while we purchase 200 slices of cheese (two per sandwich) each week at a cost of $13.00. Initially this task took over an hour, but now the men only spend about 30 minutes each Friday afternoon slapping cheese between two slices of bread.

Depending on the ability level of your participants, the job can be divided into several simple tasks along an assembly line to completion. Add extra meaning to this project by taking the men on a short field trip to the local shelter where they can actually meet the individuals who receive the food.

Write to Officials

Assist the men in writing a letter to a local member of Congress, mayor, newspaper editor, or other prominent figure about something that is important to them. During a current events discussion, our men's group became very concerned about the local increase in crime and had their own thoughts on what should be done. We wrote a letter and sent it to the mayor. The men felt so good about what they had done that they now want to write to the President!

Hold a Business Meeting

Set up a formal table arrangement where the men can sit and discuss issues that affect their lives. This may be very similar to "Resident Council" meetings, but should pertain only to the men and their interests. Discuss purchases of items men might enjoy. Discuss future activities, meals, and personal issues that concern men.

Plant a Garden

Involve the men in every aspect, from the planning stages to the planting to the daily care of a garden. Whenever possible, the garden should be raised off the ground in boxes at approximately waist height. Older individuals can become easily discouraged with all the bending and kneeling involved with an in-ground garden. Raise vegetables that can be consumed by the men and their peers, donated to worthwhile organizations, or actually sold for profit.

Share Oral Histories

Ask the men to share their life histories with school children. Contact a local school or church group to see if they are interested in interacting with a group of older men. The children can learn a lot about 20th century American history and the men feel good about sharing their experiences. You can assist by providing yearbooks and personal pictures whenever possible. Meet with the children in advance and give them tips on how to interact with the men. You might suggest the types of questions they could ask.

Give Out Jobs

Plan small, individual jobs according to past work and interests. Put someone in charge of watering plants in the facility, raising the flag each morning, assisting with the facility newsletter, opening and sorting the mail, delivering mail to residents/participants, greeting new residents/participants, or assisting those who are less able.

Examine Cars

If the men are interested in automobiles, find an old vehicle and park it in the facility parking lot. Depending on the ability of the men, they will probably spend some time discussing what can be done to improve the vehicle and others may even want to try their hand at it.

Care for Pets

Purchase a pet just for the men. Have the men decide in their business meeting if it is to be a hamster, guinea pig, or other small creature. The men, with your assistance, can divide up the tasks such as feeding, cleaning the cage, or just keeping an eye on the animal. Focusing on another living being provides purpose in life and keeps individuals from focusing on their own difficulties.

Chapter 2

Intergenerational Programming

When I first approached my men's group with the idea of interacting with children in a nearby preschool, the response was less than enthusiastic. Many thought a relationship between old men and little children would seem forced or unnatural. One man even blurted out, "My kids are grown! Why would I want to do that?"

As I thought about similar programming I had done in the past with mixed groups, I realized it was often the women who felt most comfortable with children. However, I was also convinced that men benefited a great deal from such interaction. I pressed on.

Our first "get-together" with the children lasted only 15 minutes. I think the men were more uncomfortable than the children. We sang some familiar songs and got to know each other. When it was time to leave, two five-year-olds unexpectedly climbed onto a man's lap and gave him a hug. From that moment on, our men never again had to be pushed into a visit with the children. In fact, it's one of the best things we do!

Helpful Tips to Remember

1. If the children are young (4-8 years), keep the visits relatively short: no longer than 25 minutes initially. Lengthen only if both the men and children indicate a desire to spend more time with each other.

2. Do not engage in activity involving lots of noise or running around. This will agitate those with dementia.

3. Every activity should appeal to both children and adults. Some of the men may not have spent a great deal of time playing with their own children and may feel uncomfortable playing games with someone else's children.

4. Try to have approximately the same number of children as adults. It is best to limit the entire group to 20 individuals.

Seasonal Ideas for Interactions with Young Children

Your First Meeting

Once you have introduced the idea to the men's group, schedule a brief visit between yourself and the children. During that visit, you can refer to the men as being like their grandfathers, men who want to share some games and songs with them. Ask the children to talk about their own grandfathers or grandparents. Explain that both groups can learn a lot from each other. Then allow the children to express any concerns or ask questions.

Ask the children to sing a favorite song from school. Then lead the entire group in a song that everyone knows, such as "You Are My Sunshine," "Bicycle Built for Two," or "She'll Be Comin' Round the Mountain." Can the children imagine these men being five or six years old? Present childhood pictures of the men (which you obtained earlier) and see if the children can guess which picture belongs to which man. Encourage the men to relate any special memories of childhood.

At the close, serve a snack. If they are willing, ask each child to deliver the snack to a new friend. Just before the children leave, teach everyone a simple goodbye song that can be sung at each gathering. The one below is sung to the tune of "Good Night, Ladies":

> Goodbye, my friends,
> Goodbye, my friends,
> Goodbye, my friends,
> I hope to see you soon!

Winter Fun

Before the children arrive, give each man a winter sticker to hand to a child. This encourages interaction from the start. Once the children have received their little gifts and are seated, lead the group in singing "Jingle Bells." Has anyone has ever ridden in a one-horse sleigh? How did they keep warm? Show a picture of a sleigh. Encourage the men and children to discuss what they like (or dislike) about snow.

Tell the children that if they really want it to snow, they should close their eyes tight and say, "Let it snow!" Once the children have done this, ask them to repeat it three times. This, of course, will lead you into the singing of "Let it Snow, Let it Snow, Let it Snow." The men can sing the song, while you direct the children in singing the "Let it Snow" parts. Finally, if the men are able, show everyone how to cut simple snowflakes from folded white paper. The men and children can assist each other in the cutting. Snowflakes can then be hung at the windows for a winter wonderland look.

Valentine's Day

Before the gathering, cut out enough large hearts from construction paper so that there will be one heart for each child. If the children are young, each heart should be a different color. Cut the hearts in half in various ways so that they fit back together like a puzzle. Give each man one half of a heart and hide the other half somewhere in the room.

Once the children arrive and are seated, ask them to sing "Skidamarink" or a similar Valentine's Day song to the group. Then, lead the men in singing "Let Me Call You Sweetheart." Tell the children that there are a lot of broken hearts in the room that need fixing. Invite them to search the room for a half of a heart and then match it with the correct half that a man is holding. When they find the correct man, they should wish him a happy Valentine's Day! End the gathering by serving Valentine cookies.

The Smell of Springtime

Prepare for this meeting by gathering 10-15 different items, each with a distinctive odor. Put each item in a small cup with lid so that it cannot be identified. Suggestions for items: coffee, cinnamon, garlic, toothpaste, onion, lemon, peanut butter, perfume, chocolate, or vinegar. Encourage the men and children to assist each other in identifying the items just by using their sense of smell. Afterwards, discuss memories the smells evoke. Lead the group in singing springtime songs such as "Take Me Out to the Ball Game," or "You Are My Sunshine."

Make Your Own Ice Cream Sundae

This is perfect for a hot summer day and involves less clean-up if done outside. Line a table with all the fixings for a great ice cream sundae, such as chocolate sauce, nuts, cherries, etc. Hand each child and adult a dish of vanilla ice cream and let them work together in creating the most delicious ice cream sundae around. You might want to alert the teachers ahead of time that this will be messy, but lots of fun! Then lead the group in singing "In the Good Old Summertime." Ask children and adults to name their favorite vacation spot.

Independence Day Celebration

In preparation for this gathering, find 10-15 items that are distinctly red, white, or blue or that are patriotic in nature (red candles, blue streamers, a flag, white ribbon, red shoes, etc.). Lay the items on a tray and cover with a cloth.

As the children arrive for the gathering, the men can give each child a little flag sticker. Discuss July 4th celebrations past and present. Reveal the tray and discuss each red, white, or blue item on the tray. Then cover the tray and see how many items the group can remember. In most cases, the children's memories will be much better than their adult counterparts. This is where you can really encourage interaction. The children can whisper items to the men or help each other with the answers. End the gathering by singing "America the Beautiful," "The Star Spangled Banner," or "This Land Is Your Land."

Autumn Apples

In preparation for this gathering, you should have a portable burner, large pot with hot, melted caramel, and enough apples and popsicle sticks for each child. Before the children arrive, push a popsicle stick into the top of each apple.

Once everyone is seated, tell the group the story of Johnny Appleseed. Hold up a big, red apple for everyone to see and smell. Ask the children if they can say the word "no." Then ask them to repeat it three times. (They'll love that!) This will lead you into the singing of "Don't Sit Under the Apple Tree." The men can sing the verses while the children shout the "no, no, no!" line. Finally, pair each child with an adult and have them help each other dip an apple into the hot caramel, swirl it, and place it on any aluminum foil surface to harden. The children can then take the caramel apples back with them for snack.

CAUTION: This is a somewhat hazardous activity where you need to be alert at ALL times so that neither the children nor the men burn themselves on the hot pot or burner.

Holiday Party

This can be celebrated at Thanksgiving or any time during December. Have the group sing songs such as "Over the River and Through the Woods," "Jingle

Intergenerational Programming

Bells," "We Wish You a Merry Christmas," "Rudolph the Red-nosed Reindeer," "Winter Wonderland," or "White Christmas." Ask the children and adults to share ideas of what they are thankful for. The men can present holiday gifts to the children such as coloring books or small boxes of crayons. The children can give the men holiday cards they have made in their classroom. If appropriate, invite Santa Claus. Celebrate with holiday cookies and punch.

Interacting with Older Children

1. Ask the children to read to the men individually. The men, in return, can assist with the reading and act as a sort of tutor.

2. The children can interview the men and write a life history. For men with more progressed memory loss, provide the children with specific questions that you know the men can answer. Otherwise, this project could serve to embarrass or frustrate the men involved.

3. Use the gathering as an opportunity for the children to learn firsthand about recent American history. Bring in pictures and have the men discuss, for example, their adventures in World War II, their memories of Babe Ruth, or their first plane flight.

4. Play word games or crossword puzzles, with children and adults working as teams.

5. Ask the children to bring in their pets to share with the men.

6. Use the gathering as an opportunity for the children to learn about occupations. Ask each man to describe his work life. Use pictures and props as much as possible.

7. Talk about fads (swallowing goldfish, flagpole sitting) and compare with what the teenagers are doing today.

8. Pull out a large map and encourage the men to discuss their travels. Where have they lived? Who has traveled the farthest? Ask the men to share their travel adventures with the children, and vice versa.

Chapter 3

Man and His Newspaper

In recent years, news stories have become increasingly bold in their reporting of controversial issues concerning men and their relationships to women. Newspaper headlines often scream of sexual harassment, date rape, or women's choice issues. At first, I approached these topics cautiously with the group. After all, these men were from a distant, more proper generation. Wouldn't they feel uncomfortable discussing such issues, especially with a woman?

To my surprise, the men were anxious to discuss changes in male-female relationships. While the specific issue was modern, conflicts between men and women are as old as time. The men welcomed an opportunity to debate with a woman those issues they had never quite understood about the opposite sex. While their dementia limited a very detailed discussion, the men felt full of purpose and conviction. Their opinions were validated. They were able to put their past in perspective and to discuss changes in the world today. In doing so, the current events discussion proved interesting, educational, and fun!

For many men, a cup of coffee with the morning paper was a daily ritual. The discussion of current events in a men's group serves as a natural carryover from life itself, and the benefits are numerous:

1. The discussion of current events serves as an appropriate form of orientation to date, time, and place.

2. With the selection of controversial or unusual topics, current events are useful tools for extended group conversation.

3. News stories are wonderful introductions for reminiscing. Compare today's life-styles with those of fifty years ago.

4. News of others who are less fortunate can lead to worthwhile projects and volunteer work.

5. Reading the news can be entertaining and uplifting. If you search hard enough, you can find both humorous stories and those about good people doing good things.

How to Succeed in Current Events Discussion with Men

1. Use the discussion to announce the date, season of year, next holiday, and weather conditions.

2. Don't put the group to sleep by reading the entire article word-for-word. Overall story lines can be related in two or three sentences. Make it basic enough for everyone to follow, but interesting enough to peak their curiosity.

3. While personalities differ widely, men are usually less interested in the "Dear Abby" columns, the gossipy discussions of famous personalities, the fashion section, and the horoscope.

4. When selecting articles to discuss, primarily stick to local and national headlines, the travel section, and the sports page. Find controversial issues that elicit discussion.

5. Relate interesting stories that pertain to men, such as the birthday of the Boy Scouts or a celebration honoring veterans from World War II.

6. Use other resources to enhance your story. If you are discussing the President, bring in a picture of him or of the White House. If you are discussing changes in the schools, bring in an apple or a picture of a one-room schoolhouse.

7. Avoid morbid, senseless topics. Those with dementia will also be less interested in money issues, intricate business dealings, remote world events, modern technology (fax machines or computer games), and modern issues which have little bearing on the past.

8. Always use the discussion of current events as an opportunity to reminisce. The questions below may help to encourage discussion:

   · How would you feel if you were a part of this story?

   · Would this type of incident have occurred when you were a child? Why or why not?

   · Would you like to be on the jury?

   · What should be the punishment for the criminal?

   · Why did this happen? Does this reflect positive or negative changes in society?

   · Does this remind you of incidents in your past? Is history repeating itself?

Annual Events to Add Spark to Your Discussions

January

1st: New Year's Day. The Mummers strut down Broad Street in their famous Philadelphia parade.

4th: Annual Trivia Day.

8th: Women's Day in Greece. Men do the housework and look after the children while the women relax.

9th: Birthday of 37th U.S. president Richard Nixon, born 1913.

12th: Birthday of boxer Joe Frazier, born 1944.

15th: Birthday of civil rights leader, Martin Luther King, Jr., born 1929.

February

2nd: Groundhog Day. If the animal sees his shadow, winter will continue for six more weeks.

12th: Birthday of the 16th U.S. president Abraham Lincoln, born 1809.

14th: Valentine's Day.

22nd: Birthday of the 1st U.S. president George Washington, born 1732.

27th: Birthday of actress Elizabeth Taylor, born 1932.

March

1st: National Pig Day.

11th: Birthday of orchestra leader Lawrence Welk, born 1903.

17th: St. Patrick's Day.

20th: First day of spring.

26th: Annual "Make Up Your Own Holiday" Day.

30th: Annual Doctor's Day (since 1842).

April

1st: April Fool's Day.

7th: United Nations World Health Day (since 1948).

9th: Winston Churchill Day. This marks the date Churchill was made an honorary U.S. citizen.

15th: Income tax due this day.

30th: National Honesty Day.

May

1st: Loyalty Day (since 1959) and Law Day (since 1958).

2nd: Roberts' Rules of Order Day.

3rd: Annual Lumpy Rug Day. To honor those who sweep difficult issues under the rug.

6th: The date that marks the halfway point of spring.

8th: Annual "No Socks" Day.

15th: Police Memorial Day.

18th: "Visit Your Relatives" Day.

30th: Traditional Decoration Day or Memorial Day.

June

6th: National Yo-yo Day.

14th: Flag Day.

21st: First day of summer.

July

1st: Canada Day.

2nd: Date that marks the halfway point of the year. At noon, 182 1/2 days have passed and 182 1/2 remain.

4th: U.S. Independence Day.

12th: Birthday of Mr. Television, Milton Berle, born 1908.

13th: Muslim New Year.

28th: Birthday of former First Lady, Jacqueline Kennedy Onassis, born 1929.

August

4th: Coast Guard Day (since 1970).

5th: National Mustard Day.

7th: Date that marks the halfway point of summer.

15th: National Relaxation Day.

19th: National Aviation Day (since 1939).

23rd: Birthday of actor/dancer Gene Kelly, born 1912.

September

4th: Annual Newspaper Carrier Day. The hiring of the first newsboy happened this day in 1833.

7th: "Neither Rain Nor Snow" Day. Honors the nation's letter carriers.

13th: Birthday of actress Claudette Colbert, born 1905.

15th: Annual "Bed Check" Day. Designed as a date to check your mattress for signs of wear.

15th: "Respect for the Aged" Day in Japan.

16th: Independence Day in Mexico.

17th: Citizenship Day.

18th: Birthday of the U.S. Air Force (since 1947).

22nd: Birthday of the ice cream cone, invented in 1903.

22nd: First day of autumn.

29th: Birthday of actor/singer Gene Autry, born 1907.

October

4th: "Ten-Four Day." This is the fourth day of the tenth month of the year. It is also a phrase used on two-way radios, as in "Ten-four, good buddy." It is an affirmative reply.

10th: Birthday of actress Helen Hayes, born 1900.

12th: Traditional Columbus Day.

13th: Birthday of the White House, 1600 Pennsylvania Ave., Washington, D.C. The cornerstone was laid on October 13, 1792.

14th: Annual "Be Bald and Be Free" Day.

15th: National Grouch Day.

24th: United Nations Day, founded on October 24, 1945.

27th: Annual Navy Day.

31st: Halloween.

November

5th: Birthday of actor Roy Rogers, born 1912.

8th: Birthday of actress Katharine Hepburn, born 1909.

10th: Birthday of the U.S. Marine Corps, established 1775.

11th: Traditional Armistice Day or Veterans Day. Celebrates the armistice of World War I, 1918.

December

9th: Birthday of actor Douglas Fairbanks, Jr., born 1909.

10th: Human Rights Day. Celebrates the anniversary of the adoption of the United Nations' "Universal Declaration of Human Rights."

10th: Birthday of actress Dorothy Lamour, born 1914.

21st: First day of winter.

25th: Christmas.

26th: Boxing Day in Canada and the United Kingdom. Originally, this holiday began as the day when Christmas boxes were given to those who provided regular public services, such as the postman and the lamplighter.

31st: "Make Up Your Mind" Day.

31st: New Year's Eve.

Chapter 4

Reminiscing

Almost every week in our men's group, a brilliant, 84-year-old scientist recounts fondly the story of his first day of school. He was a mere four years old and got into a fistfight with an older boy in the schoolyard. He must have won that battle because the memory has stayed with him for 80 years! More than his many professional awards or travels around the world, the memory of his first day of school helps define him and give his life meaning.

One of the most effective tools in activity programming with older adults (especially those with dementia) is the use of reminiscing: allowing participants to freely discuss their past. Reminiscing serves to validate life experiences and puts the past in perspective. By recalling the past, participants are saying, "This is what I did and who I was. My life was important to others. These events helped shape who I am today." Such discussions are sometimes a safe outlet for exploring feelings concerning past events.

Reminiscing is a pleasant and non-threatening experience. Those with dementia often lose short-term memory, while their recall of the distant past remains amazingly intact. Discussion of this past can increase feelings of security and create a common bond among group members. Anxiety and agitation are reduced when participants are not focusing on current problems and disabilities.

Helpful Tips for Conducting Reminiscing Discussions

1. Listen to what the participant is saying. Focus on memories which were important to that individual, not what might have been important or fascinating to you.

2. Validate memories and feelings. Do not dismiss sad or angry feelings. This is often referred to as active listening. When the group leader responds with statements such as, "I can understand how you felt," or "You must have been frightened when that happened," the individual feels as though his emotions are important. This type of validation helps to build trust and a sense of security between the group leader and group members.

3. Use props to enhance the discussion. Pictures, distinctive smells, objects, and related music bring memories to life and are nearly essential when

working with those who are cognitively impaired.

4. Do not ask direct questions that are too difficult to answer or may frustrate the group members. Ask leading questions that do not require specific answers. Instead of asking, "How many children did you have," you might say, "I'll bet children added a lot of excitement to your home life! Can you tell us anything special about your family?"

5. Don't use reminiscing just for specific discussion groups. Incorporate memories into every aspect of your activity program. Sing old songs, remember Grandma's kitchen while cooking, or discuss memories of the old general store while playing checkers.

Following this are eight topics for reminiscing with older men. Memory objects or "props" are suggested for each topic to help encourage memories and enhance discussion.

Topics

Men's Clothing and Accessories, p. 16
World War II, p. 18
The Great Depression, p. 20
Movies and Entertainment, p. 22
Radio, p. 24
Automobiles, p. 26
Planes and Trains, p. 28
Occupations, p. 30

Reminiscing

Men's Clothing and Accessories

Suggested Props

Pocket watch
Money clip
Derby hat
Suspenders
Bow tie
Old Sears and Roebuck catalog

Picture Sources

Eldergames - "How Things Have Changed: Fashion"

Time-Life Books - *This Fabulous Century, 1930-1940* contains a Depression-era shopping list of men's clothing

Facts to Share

1. In the early part of the century, boy's shirts were called "blouses." They were full cut with an elastic waistband.

2. In the 1928 presidential election, Alfred E. Smith's campaign symbol was a familiar article of clothing, a brown derby hat.

3. Fashionable men's trousers in the early 1920s were a full 22 inches wide at the leg cuff.

4. Men's shirts in the 1930s often did not have attached collars. An expensive silk shirt in that era cost $4.48. A flannel shirt was sold for $2.00.

5. In 1933, a man's pullover sweater cost less than $2.00. A wool suit was only $10.50 and a silk necktie could be purchased for 55 cents.

Trivia

1. In the early part of the 20th century, what was used to keep men's socks from sagging? Answer: Garters

2. What was the name for knee-length pants worn by young boys? Answer: Knickerbockers or "knickers"

3. What was used to hold up trousers before belts? Answer: Suspenders

4. A long, military-style coat with a belt is called what? Answer: Trench coat

5. A suit with two rows of buttons is called what? Answer: Double breasted

6. What is the slang term for winter underwear that covers the entire body? Answer: Longjohns

7. What were "plus-fours"? Answer: Extra wide knickers often worn when golfing

8. What material were Panama hats often made of? Answer: Straw. They were summer hats.

9. Another name for a military uniform is what? Answer: Fatigues

10. A baggy, oversized suit worn by fashionable teenagers in the 1940s was called what? Answer: A zoot suit

11. Name the cloth or leather covering for the top of a shoe. Answer: Spat

12. A stiff felt hat with a dome-shaped crown and narrow brim is called what? Answer: Derby hat

13. Describe "Oxford bags," often worn by men in the 1920s. Answer: Wide-legged trousers

14. Where do you wear a cummerbund? Answer: Around the waist on formal occasions

15. What is a beret? Answer: A hat of French origin, often made of felt, and worn tilted to the side of the head

16. Why would a man wear a toupee? Answer: To cover a bald spot or to change the appearance of his hair. A toupee is a false hair piece for men.

17. How was a pocket watch attached to the trousers? Answer: By a chain or a fob

18. Describe a man's bathing suit in the early 1920s. Answer: A two-piece garment with trunks and a sleeveless shirt

19. What is an ascot? Answer: A decorative neck scarf, tied loosely under the chin

20. What is a "four-in-hand"? Answer: A long necktie that is tied in a slip knot

Questions for Discussion

1. Did you ever own a pocket watch? Who gave you the watch? Was it on a special occasion?

2. Do you recall wearing a bathing suit that covered your chest? Describe it. Was it made of a heavy material? What do you think of today's bathing suits?

3. In the past, men always wore hats outdoors. Did you have a hat you especially enjoyed wearing? Describe your favorite hat. Why do you think hats have gone out of style?

4. Describe the clothing you wore as a boy. Did you wear knickers? At what age could a young man begin wearing full-length pants?

5. If you were in the military, describe your uniform. What did you dislike most about military clothing? What clothing did you purchase first when you returned to civilian life?

World War II

Suggested Props

Soldiers' emblems
Recording of swing music
Tin foil (reminiscent of scrap drives)
Coffee grounds (reminiscent of rationing)

Picture Sources

Time-Life Books - *This Fabulous Century, 1940-1950*

Eldergames - "Flashbacks: Famous Faces and Events"

Facts to Share

1. M&Ms were first produced in 1940 for the U.S. military. The candy would melt in the mouth and not stain the uniform!

2. During World War II, Jack Benny's violin was auctioned for $1 million to raise money for the purchase of war bonds.

3. In 1945, a B-25 aircraft crashed into the Empire State building, killing 13 people.

4. In 1945, Adolf Hitler and Eva Braun were married for one day.

5. In the summer of 1942, President Roosevelt had four sons in active duty: James, Elliot, Franklin, and John.

6. The G.I. bill of rights, a veterans benefit bill, was passed in 1944.

Trivia

1. Name the man who became prime minister of England in 1940. Answer: Winston Churchill

2. During World War II, Americans grew vegetables in their gardens for the war effort. What were these gardens called? Answer: Victory gardens

3. Where were the Allied planes when they flew over "the hump"? Answer: Over the Himalaya Mountains

4. What powerful weapon was developed as a result of the Manhattan Project, led by Dr. Robert Oppenheimer? Answer: The atomic bomb

5. Name the Hawaiian port city that was attacked by the Japanese on December 7, 1941. Answer: Pearl Harbor

6. Was Stalin a tall man? Answer: No (He was only 5'5".)

7. What organization was formed in 1945 in hopes of ensuring world peace? Its headquarters is located in New York City. Answer: The United Nations

8. During World War II, George Patton created an uproar by publicly doing what to two soldiers? Answer: He slapped them

9. Name the four-wheel drive, all-purpose vehicle used as ground transportation during World War II. Answer: Jeep

10. Who was Private Eddie Slovik? Answer: The first U. S. soldier to be executed for desertion since the Civil War

11. Name President Roosevelt's dog who sparked controversy during the 1944 election. Answer: Fala

12. V-E Day was on May 8, 1945. What do the initials V-E stand for? Answer: Victory in Europe

13. What famous, symbolic event occurred at Iwo Jima after U.S. troops won back the island from Japan? Answer: The American flag was raised

14. For those in the military, what is "Stars and Stripes"? Answer: A daily newspaper published for men and women in the armed forces

15. Did U.S. forces ever invade northern Africa during World War II? Answer: Yes (on November 16, 1942)

16. What were U-boats? Answer: German submarines

17. What was Audie Murphy's occupation during World War II? Answer: War correspondent

18. During World War II, the U.S. tested atomic bombs on which Pacific Island (which later also became the name of a skimpy women's bathing suit)? Answer: Bikini Island

19. Where are the "shores of Tripoli," as mentioned in the Marine song? Answer: In Libya

20. Which World War II general was known for smoking a corncob pipe? Answer: Douglas MacArthur

Questions for Discussion

1. Did you serve in the military during World War II? If so, in what branch of the military? Were you drafted or did you volunteer? Where were you stationed? Was this your first time away from home? Describe your feelings.

2. What was the mood of the United States during World War II? Was patriotism running high?

3. If you were on the "home front" during the war, what did you do? Did you grow a victory garden? Did you help with scrap drives? What did you collect?

4. Do you remember where you were when you heard that Pearl Harbor had been attacked? Did you believe the story at first? How did you react?

5. If you were in the military, describe how your hometown welcomed you home after the war. Was there a parade? Were you treated as a hero? How did you feel?

6. How did your experiences during World War II change your life or change you as a person?

Reminiscing

The Great Depression

Suggested Props

Apples
Potatoes
Money
Ticker tape

Picture Sources

Time-Life Books - *This Fabulous Century, 1930-1940*

Eldergames - "Flashback: Famous Faces and Events"

Facts to Share

1. On the day of the stock market crash, October 29, 1929, $30 billion was lost.

2. By 1933, nearly 14 million Americans were unemployed.

3. In one year, so many homeless individuals sought shelter in railroad box cars, that the Southern Pacific Railroad added extra cars to accommodate the destitute. Nearly 700,000 individuals used these box cars for shelter.

4. The first woman shot by the FBI was bank robber Bonnie Parker of "Bonnie and Clyde" fame.

5. In November, 1933, a giant dust storm blew across North Dakota, burying farms and killing livestock. This was the beginning of a series of such storms that devastated Colorado, Oklahoma, and much of the Midwest. Many farmers packed up their few remaining belongings and headed for California in search of a better life.

Trivia

1. What tragedy struck Charles and Anne Morrow Lindbergh in the early 1930s? Answer: Their baby was kidnapped and murdered

2. Which U.S. president ran for election promising a "new deal for the American people"? Answer: Franklin D. Roosevelt

3. In 1933, what did President Roosevelt say was the only thing we have to fear? Answer: Fear itself

4. Where was "Wrong Way" Corrigan supposedly heading when he landed in Dublin, Ireland? Answer: California

5. What happened to the airship, the Hindenburg, over Lakehurst, New Jersey, in 1937? Answer: It exploded

6. What happened to the nation's banks on March 4, 1933, President Hoover's last day in office? Answer: The nation's entire banking system collapsed

7. Who was Aimee Semple McPherson? Answer: A controversial and outspoken evangelist (often known for her "angel" pose)

8. What fruit did unemployed people sell on street corners? Answer: Apples

9. What was a "Hoover blanket"? Answer: Newspaper used to cover a homeless person on a park bench

10. Franklin Roosevelt's wife was very influential in politics. She even wrote a daily newspaper column entitled "My Day." What was her name? Answer: Eleanor Roosevelt

11. The CCC was part of the New Deal legislation, working on conservation and reforestation. What did the initials stand for? Answer: Civilian Conservation Corps

12. What disease crippled President Franklin Roosevelt? Answer: Polio

13. In 1934, what gangster was considered "Public Enemy #1"? Answer: John Dillinger

14. This mayor of New York City during the 1930s was nicknamed "The Little Flower." Can you name him? Answer: Fiorello La Guardia

15. What bird was the symbol of the National Recovery Administration (NRA)? Answer: The (blue) eagle

16. What devastating event occurred in Johnstown, Pennsylvania in 1936? Answer: A flood nearly destroyed the city

17. The Hoover Dam (later renamed the Boulder Dam) was completed in 1936. It rests between Nevada and what other state? Answer: Arizona

18. In President Franklin Roosevelt's New Deal legislation, what did the letters T.V.A. stand for? Answer: Tennessee Valley Authority

19. What was Franklin Roosevelt's "Amberjack II"? Answer: His sailboat

20. The Empire State Building opened in 1931 in what Eastern city? Answer: New York City

Questions for Discussion

1. How did you hear about the stock market crash in 1929? How did the crash affect you?

2. Did you or a member of your family lose a job during the Depression? Describe what you did to conserve money and family resources. Were there many "meatless" meals?

3. During a time when money was in short supply, what did you do for entertainment? Did you play games at home? Did you go to the matinee movies for a dime?

4. If you lived in a city during this time, did you see men selling apples on street corners? Did hoboes or tramps ever knock on your door, asking for a handout? How did you feel about this?

Movies and Entertainment

Suggested Props

Ticket stub
Popcorn
Old movie poster

Picture Sources

Eldergames - "Flashback to Hollywood's Golden Age" (Musical and Comedy Stars; Dramatic Stars)

Time-Life Books - *This Fabulous Century, 1930-1940*

Facts to Share

1. During World War II, some movie theaters asked kids to bring scrap metal instead of purchasing a ticket. This war effort backfired when some children actually donated their father's tools or their mother's good pots and pans.

2. The most elaborate and expensive movie of the 1930s was "Gone With the Wind" starring Vivien Leigh and Clark Gable.

3. In 1934, American Roman Catholic Bishops founded the National League of Decency. Their efforts banned long kisses, adultery, double beds, and even nude babies from Hollywood films.

4. Between 1947 and 1950, nearly 2,000 drive-in movie theaters were built across the country.

Trivia

1. Name the 1930s comic strip hero who was kidnapped to the planet Mongo by the evil "Ming the Merciless." Answer: Flash Gordon

2. In "Tarzan the Apeman," who was Tarzan's mate? Answer: Jane

3. How did comedian Will Rogers die? Answer: Killed in a plane crash with Wiley Post in Alaska

4. In the movie "She Done Him Wrong," who invited Cary Grant to "come up sometime and see me"? Answer: Mae West

5. The movie "Public Enemy" had a shocking scene in which James Cagney shoved what fruit into Mae Clark's face? Answer: Grapefruit

6. Who was known as the blonde bombshell in the 1930s? Answer: Jean Harlow

7. With what 1930s comic strip would you associate the evil "Killer Kane" and "Ardala," disintegrator guns, and the solar scouts? Answer: Buck Rogers

8. What tall building in New York City did King Kong climb? Answer: The Empire State Building

9. Name the "straight shooter" cowboy whose Wonder Horse was named "Tony." Answer: Tom Mix

10. Tess Truehart was engaged to what 1930s comic strip detective? Answer: Dick Tracy

11. What cowboy used "Back In the Saddle Again" as his theme song? Answer: Gene Autry

12. What comedy team did the famous "Who's On First" routine? Answer: Abbott and Costello

13. Groucho, Chico, Harpo, Zeppo, and Gummo were a comedy team better known as what? Answer: The Marx Brothers

14. In 1935, this well-known dance team starred in the movie "Top Hat." His name was Fred Astaire. Can you name his partner? Answer: Ginger Rogers

15. Al Jolson starred in the "Jazz Singer," the first movie of what distinction? Answer: The first full-length "talkie"

16. The first widely-syndicated comic strip of the 1930s featured Dagwood Bumstead and his wife. What was her name? Answer: Blondie

17. Name the leading man paired with Katharine Hepburn in nine films, starting with "Woman of the Year." Answer: Spencer Tracy

18. What was Fred Waring's profession? Answer: Leader of a 70-man band known as the Pennsylvanians

19. The biggest box office star in 1938 was a curly-haired little girl. Can you name her? Answer: Shirley Temple

20. Name Little Orphan Annie's dog. Answer: Sandy

Questions for Discussion

1. Did you look forward to Saturday afternoon matinees? Some theaters gave away door prizes. Did you ever win a prize? What were some of the items given away?

2. Did you read comic books as a youngster? Who were your favorite comic heroes?

3. Do you enjoy westerns? Who was your favorite cowboy, John Wayne, Tom Mix, or Gene Autry?

4. Do you remember silent movies? Do you recall the organ player at the front of the theater? How did movies change when sound was introduced? Were they better?

Reminiscing

Radio

Suggested Props

An old radio
Earphones
Microphone
Recordings of old radio shows
Recordings of music from the 1920s, 1930s, and 1940s

Facts to Share

1. In 1920, radios were wireless with individual headphones for listeners. Only later, when horn-shaped loud speakers were developed, could families enjoy listening together.

2. The nation's first radio station, KDKA in Pittsburgh, made history on November 1, 1920, by broadcasting the Harding-Cox presidential returns.

3. Sales of radios in 1920 reached $2 million; in 1929, sales topped $600 million.

4. Radios began to be installed in automobiles in the early 1930s.

Trivia

1. Name George Burns' wife and comic partner. Answer: Gracie Allen

2. Walter Winchell began his 1930s radio show by saying "Good Evening, Mr. and Mrs." what? Answer: America

3. What instrument did Benny Goodman play? Answer: Clarinet

4. Name the radio star who sang "When the Moon Comes Over the Mountain." Answer: Kate Smith

5. Franklin D. Roosevelt communicated with the American public over the radio in a series of what? Answer: Fireside chats

6. What two words did President Roosevelt use to begin each of his Fireside chats? Answer: "My Friends"

7. How did Major Bowes tell contestants that their time was up on his Amateur Hour? Answer: He rang a gong

8. The NBC Jello program on Sunday evenings featured comedian Jack Benny playing what instrument? Answer: Violin

9. Who was Charlie McCarthy, featured on the Chase and Sanborn Hour, Sunday evenings at 8:00 p.m.? Answer: Edgar Bergen's wooden dummy

10. On Sunday, October 30, 1938, Orson Welles broadcast a program about aliens landing in New Jersey, which caused a panic among Americans. What was the name of the show? Answer: "War of the Worlds"

11. In the early 1940s, what did Ray Noble do on radio's Chase and Sanborn hour? Answer: He led the orchestra

12. Name the dramatic radio show that starred a masked cowboy with a companion named Tonto. Answer: "The Lone Ranger"

13. In 1940, what evening of the week did "Time" magazine name as the most popular for radio listeners? Answer: Sunday

14. Who lived with Fibber McGee at 79 Wistful Vista? Answer: Molly

15. In April, 1945, a minute of silence was observed over the radio marking the death of what well-known American? Answer: President Franklin Roosevelt

16. Clifton Fadiman was the moderator of a popular radio show entitled, "Information —" what? Answer: Please

17. "The Adventures of the Nelson Family" began on radio in 1944. What were the couple's first names? Answer: Ozzie and Harriet

18. On a popular 1940s radio series, the character "Archie" was the manager of what tavern? Answer: Duffy's Tavern

19. What was unique about the orchestra on Phil Spitalny's radio show, "The House of Charm"? Answer: It was an "all-girl" orchestra

20. Name the popular radio personality who was known as the "man with the barefoot voice." Answer: Arthur Godfrey

Questions for Discussion

1. How did the introduction of radio change your family life? Did your family sit together in the living room to listen? Did you look forward to certain shows?

2. Did you ever worry that your children were listening to too much radio?

3. Did you listen to the "War of the Worlds" broadcast in 1938? Did the broadcast frighten you? Describe the panic that spread throughout the country that night.

4. Who were your favorite comics on radio? What type of shows did you enjoy?

5. Did you have a radio in your automobile?

6. What music did you like to hear on the radio? Did you ever listen to the Grand Ole Opry on WJM? The Metropolitan Opera broadcasts?

Reminiscing

Automobiles

Suggested Props

Driving gloves
Model cars
Books with pictures of old automobiles
  (see Resource List)

Related Movie

"Tucker, the Man and His Dream" - This film relates the true story of a man who started an American automobile company in 1948. (See Facts to Share #5.)

Facts to Share

1. Before 1920, most cars had open bodies, which meant you would get wet and cold in bad weather.

2. Many early cars had a split windshield. The upper half could be opened outward for ventilation.

3. In the 1920s, special care had to be taken so the car's radiator wouldn't freeze overnight. In winter, car owners would drain the radiator or cover it with a warm blanket.

4. Balloon tires were introduced in 1922, providing a much smoother ride on rough roads.

5. Shortly after World War II, the Tucker automobile factory opened in the U.S. with the dream of building safer and more powerful cars. Unfortunately, only 50 Tucker Torpedoes were ever produced before the factory was closed due to financial difficulties. Powered by a Sikorsky helicopter engine, the Tucker Torpedo is a valuable collector's item today.

6. At the 1939 New York World's Fair, futuristic automobiles of 1960 were envisioned as radio controlled with rear engines and air conditioning.

7. In 1940, the Ford automobile factory contained the largest room in the world.

8. Prices for cars and related equipment in 1933:

   Pontiac coupe $585.00
   Chrysler sedan $995.00
   Dodge $595.00
   Studebaker $840.00
   Packard $2150.00
   Chevrolet truck $650.00
   Automobile tire $6.20
   Gasoline .... 18 cents per gallon

Trivia

1. The Model T Ford came in only one color. What was it? Answer: Black

2. What was the name for the small back seat of a car which folded down? Answer: Rumble seat

3. What kind of car has a removable roof? Answer: A convertible

4. Where was the crank on a Model T Ford inserted? Answer: In a hole just below the radiator

5. What is a "jalopy"? Answer: An old, dilapidated car

6. In the 1930s, one company cleverly used a series of six small signs along the highway to advertise its product. What was this product? Answer: Burma Shave

7. Why were early cars raised high off the ground? Answer: They required lots of clearance to avoid the mud and bumps on unpaved roads

8. Where was the nation's first all-vehicle tunnel built in 1927? Answer: In New York (the Holland Tunnel, completed in 1927)

9. How were headlights powered on early model cars? Answer: From a battery

10. Were automobiles produced in the United States during World War II? Answer: No

11. What material made up the steering wheel and the wheel spokes of the Model T Ford? Answer: Wood

12. What was the name of the footboard that was built along the outside of an automobile? Answer: The running board

13. On early cars, what were known as "suicide doors"? Answer: Doors that opened from the front. Often the wind would catch the door and it could fly open unexpectedly.

14. What country manufactured Volkswagens? Answer: Germany

15. Where can you find the Peace Bridge, built in the 1920s? Answer: On the border between the United States and Canada (near Buffalo, New York)

16. What American auto manufacturer introduced the first family station wagon in 1928? Answer: Ford

17. What is a "bald" tire? Answer: One that has no tread, causing it to slip on the road

18. President Herbert Hoover was quoted as promising a "chicken in every pot and what in every garage? Answer: A car

19. In 1931, what distinction did the Bluebird automobile hold? Answer: It was the world's most powerful automobile

20. In 1927, Volvo automobiles were first imported from what country? Answer: Sweden

Questions for Discussion

1. How did you learn to drive? How old were you at the time?

2. Do you recall your first car? Describe the car. Do you remember the purchase price of the car? How did you pay for it?

3. Did you ever crank up a car to get it started? Describe the experience.

4. Did your family enjoy Sunday drives in the country? Was this a weekly family outing? Where did you usually drive?

5. Do you remember drive-in movies? Were they popular spots to take a date? How did drive-in movies compare with theaters?

Planes and Trains

Suggested Props

Model train
Model airplane
Conductor's hat
Airlines or train ticket
Train whistle
Pictures of trains and/or planes (see Resource List or *This Fabulous Century, 1920-1930*)

Facts to Share

1. In the mid-1920s, street cars ran down the main avenues of most major cities in America. A ride usually cost 5 cents. The street cars used air brakes and were powered by electric motors.

2. In 1934, air conditioning was introduced to passenger trains, making the long rides much more comfortable. Most trains switched to diesel power by the end of the 1930s.

3. Ironically, in 1940, a portion of the elevated train tracks in New York was torn down and the scrap metal was sold to Japan!

4. For many years, night flying was considered too dangerous due to limited navigational equipment. As a result, coast-to-coast travel in 1929 was a combination of airline travel during the day and rail travel at night. The entire trip took two full days.

5. In the 1920s, the Ford Motor Company manufactured airplanes called the Stout Ford Airplanes.

Trivia

1. In what U.S. city will you find Grand Central Station? Answer: New York

2. Name the courageous pilot who flew non-stop from New York to Paris in 1927. Answer: Charles Lindbergh

3. What was the name of Charles Lindbergh's famous airplane? Answer: "The Spirit of St. Louis"

4. In railroad terminology, what was the "Iron Horse"? Answer: The huge locomotive engine

5. Why were lemons served to early airlines travelers? Answer: To help cure air sickness

6. What is the term for the railroad passenger car that included special furnishings for sleeping or night travel? Answer: Pullman car

7. What was the term for aerial shows in which early pilots performed daring stunts high above farmer's fields? Answer: Barnstorming

8. The Twentieth Century Limited passenger train traveled between two major U.S. cities. What were they? Answer: Chicago and New York

9. What is the term for the individual who serves meals and assists passengers on an airplane? Answer: Steward or stewardess (or flight attendant)

10. Who assists with luggage on a train? Answer: Porter or Red Cap

11. In politics, what was "whistle stop" campaigning? Answer: Political candidates traveled from town to town by train, often delivering speeches from the observation platform on the back of the train

12. Where do you eat meals on a train? Answer: In the dining car

13. How would you alert a trolley driver that you wanted to stop? Answer: You pulled an overhead string that rang a bell in the front

14. In the 1920s, was airmail delivered in U.S. government planes or in private aircraft? Answer: Private contractors carried the mail

15. In 1938, Howard Hughes set a record of 91 hours, 14 minutes, for flying where? Answer: Around the world

16. What is the "cowcatcher" on a railroad locomotive? Answer: An inclined frame on the front of the engine designed to remove obstacles from the tracks

17. What happened to famous aviator Amelia Earhart in 1937? Answer: She disappeared in a flight over the South Pacific

18. What new type of aircraft did Igor Sikosky develop in 1939? Answer: The helicopter

19. What was the "Spruce Goose"? Answer: A huge, wooden airplane developed by wealthy eccentric Howard Hughes. (In 1947, it was the largest plane in the world.)

20. The U. S. Air Force was formally named as a separate military service in 1947. What was it called before that time? Answer: The Army Air Corps

Questions for Discussion

1. Do you recall your first train ride? How old were you? Where did you travel? Did you sleep on the train? Describe your experience.

2. How old were you when you first flew in a plane? Were you frightened? Did you ever become air sick?

3. Did any trains run through your town? Did you ever go down to the station just to see who was getting off the train? Did anyone famous ever visit your town by train?

4. If you lived in the city, did you often travel by streetcar? Did your parents allow you to travel on the streetcar alone? Where did the streetcar take you?

5. Do you recall train excursions, often on Sunday afternoon, that took passengers outside the city to the beach, picnic grounds, or amusement park? Did you ever travel on one of these excursions? Describe the experience.

Reminiscing

Occupations

Suggested Props

Chef's hat, policeman's hat, construction worker's hat, etc.
Stethoscope
Chalk
Carpenter's tools
Typewriter
Briefcase
Textbooks
Money
Paycheck
Tie or cuff links

Facts to Share

1. Annual earnings during the Depression years:

    Physician $3382.00
    Schoolteacher $1227.00
    Steelworker $422.87
    Farmhand $216.00
    U.S. Congressman $8663.00
    Streetcar conductor ... $1040.00
    Construction worker ... $907.00
    Statistician $1820.00

2. In the mid-1800s, more than one-third of the U.S. factory labor force was made up of children. These children often worked 72 hours each week and earned as little as 11 cents per day. By 1900, 1.7 million children in the United States between 10 and 15 years of age were employed, most in mines and textile factories.

3. The country's first Labor Day was on September 5, 1882, when 10,000 workers marched in a parade up New York's Fifth Avenue. Labor Day finally became a national holiday in 1894. It's celebrated the first Monday in September.

4. President Woodrow Wilson was the first to pass federal legislation limiting child labor in 1916. The Keating-Owen Act prohibited interstate shipment of goods that had been made by children under the age of 14 or by children who had worked more than eight hours per day.

5. During the mid-1930s, American labor began to organize and fight for basic rights. For the steelworker, factory worker, or automobile assembler, wages were often very low and safety conditions even worse. Workers began to strike in huge numbers across the country. Frequently violence erupted, but by the end of the decade American workers had made great strides in improving their workplace and terms of employment.

6. As part of his New Deal legislation, Franklin Roosevelt proposed the Fair Labor Standards Act in 1938. This set an initial minimum wage of 25 cents per hour, with gradual mandated increases to 40 cents per hour. It also set the maximum work week at 40 hours, with time-and-a-half for overtime work. Once this legislation went into effect, more than 750,000 workers received an immediate increase in pay and more than a million jubilant others now had more time to spend with their families.

7. The Fair Labor Standards Act of 1938 set 16 as the minimum age for children to work in factories and it restricted children under 18 from working in hazardous conditions.

8. The Social Security Act was introduced in 1935, creating a federally-administered system of retirement payments for the nation's employed. Medical care for the elderly was added in 1965.

Trivia

1. What was Dwight D. Eisenhower's occupation before he was elected President of the United States? Answer: An army general (five-star) and Supreme Commander of Allied Forces during World War II; after that, president of Columbia University

2. What was Eleanor Roosevelt's position following her years as First Lady? Answer: Appointed to the U.S. delegation to the United Nations

3. What was the 52-20 club for servicemen following World War II? Answer: Unemployment pay for G.I.s who received $20 each week for a maximum of one year

4. Who was John L. Lewis? Answer: Powerful labor organizer, lobbyist, and strike leader during the 1930s

5. Describe a carhop's job. Answer: Delivered food and beverage to customers sitting in cars at fast food places

6. Describe a bootlegger's job. Answer: Produced and sold illegal liquor during Prohibition

7. What was Woodrow Wilson's occupation prior to becoming President of the United States? Answer: President of Princeton University and governor of New Jersey

8. What was the occupation of Bessie Smith? Answer: A blues singer (called "Empress of the Blues")

9. What was the occupation of Sinclair Lewis? Answer: Novelist

10. What position did J. Edgar Hoover hold for most of his life? Answer: Director of the Federal Bureau of Investigation

11. Describe a soda jerk's job. Answer: Served beverages and ice cream at a soda fountain

12. What was the occupation of Clarence Darrow? Answer: Lawyer

Questions for Discussion

1. Do you remember your first job? What did you do? How old were you?

2. What was your primary occupation? How did you choose this line of work?

3. Describe your most memorable "boss."

4. If you could have chosen another type of work, what would your occupation have been? Why?

5. What is more important, enjoying your profession or earning a lot of money?

6. How did you feel when you received your first paycheck?

7. Do you remember when Social Security started? How did you feel about it?

Chapter 5

Music

Music is at the heart of life itself. You would have a hard time finding someone who doesn't like to sing, at least in the shower. Music is effective in easing depression and beneficial in evoking memories and emotions. It serves to soothe agitation and anxiety and helps to create good feelings among group members. In a men's group, military songs and sports songs often serve to bond the group together in a common interest. The men have a wonderful time singing together.

Men like to sing old songs as much as women do. Old war songs, college fight songs, drinking songs, and traveling tunes are often very popular with men. And they especially like singing about women!

Listed below are some dates throughout the year which might serve as an excellent time to celebrate with music:

January 28: National Kazoo Day

February 8: Anniversary of the first opera in America, 1735, in Charleston, South Carolina

April: International Guitar Month

April 11: Barbershop Quartet Day

May, 1st Friday: International Tuba Day

July 4: National Country Music Day

September: National Piano Month

November, 1st week: American Music Week

November 6: Saxophone Day

November 6: Birthday of composer John Philip Sousa, 1854

November 22: St. Cecilia's Day (feastday of musicians)

Suggestions for Sing-alongs

Patriotic Songs

"You're in the Army Now"
"The Marine's Hymn"
"Anchors Aweigh"
"This is the Army, Mr. Jones"
"I Left My Heart At the Stage Door Canteen"
"He's A-1 in the Army and He's A-1 With Me"
"Praise the Lord and Pass the Ammunition"
"America the Beautiful"
"You're a Grand Old Flag"
"The Star Spangled Banner"

"When the Saints Go Marching In"
"My Country 'Tis of Thee"
"When Johnny Comes Marching Home"
"Yankee Doodle Boy"
"Don't Sit Under the Apple Tree"

Drinking Songs

"Show Me the Way to Go Home"
"There is a Tavern in the Town"
"Beer Barrel Polka"
"Hail, Hail, the Gang's All Here"
"Hallelujah, I'm a Bum"

Sports Songs

"Take Me Out to the Ball Game"
"Hudson High Fight Song"
"Camptown Races"
"On Wisconsin"
"Cheer, Cheer for Old Notre Dame"

Traveling Songs

"My Merry Oldsmobile"
"Chattanooga Choo Choo"
"The Sidewalks of New York"
"The Wabash Cannonball"
"The Erie Canal"
"I've Been Working on the Railroad"
"There's a Long, Long Trail"

Song Parodies

If group members are fairly high functioning, they might enjoy learning silly songs or spoofs on familiar tunes. One of the gentlemen in our group sings his state college song so often that now everyone requests it and we all know the words by heart. Following are some "silly" lyrics to three familiar tunes:

Blest Be the Tie That Binds

Blest be the tie that binds
My collar to my shirt
For underneath its silken folds
Is half an inch of dirt.

Blest be the tie that binds
My collar to my shirt
And catches the gravy from my vest
And saves it for dessert.

On Top of Old Baldy

(Tune: "On Top of Old Smokey")

On top of Old Baldy, there's hardly a hair
Just only the memory of hair that was there.

Hair parts in the middle, hair parts on the side
But parting's a sorrow when your part gets too wide.

The Man on the New Pair of Skis

(Tune: "The Man on the Flying Trapeze")

He floats down the slopes with the greatest of ease
The daring young man on the new pair of skis,
His actions are graceful, all girls he does please,
And my love he has stolen away.
This maid that I loved, she was handsome.
And I tried all I knew her to please.
But I never could please her one quarter so well
As the man on the new pair of skis.
He floats down the slopes with the greatest of class,
He misses a turn and he lands on his....(face)
His actions are graceful as the girls he does pass,
And my love he has stolen away!

Music

Chapter 6

Men and Food

Most men love to eat but not all of them feel comfortable in the kitchen. Those who have never mastered the art of cooking may feel threatened or insecure. Others may approach the project with gusto, thoroughly enjoying the experience. In the end, however, nearly everyone feels a sense of pride while savoring the delicious results.

Preparing food is a great activity for impaired adults. It does not require small or exacting actions, mistakes can be made without ruining the end result, and much of the task is repetitive (stirring, kneading, etc.). The preparation of food is activity with an obvious purpose, and when the project is completed, everyone has a great time making it disappear!

Evaluate your group before conducting a cooking activity: Who has prepared food in the past? Does anyone have a special recipe he enjoys? Which group members have never prepared food? Does anyone feel insulted by the idea of cooking? Once you have answered these questions, it's time to begin.

Select a recipe and write it in large print on a poster board. Refer to the poster board frequently so that the men focus on what they are doing. Some men may not be aware of kitchen terminology. Explain terms and tools as you go along, but don't be condescending.

Men like hearty meals with fun ingredients. Don't forget to ask them to assist with cleaning up. For many, this is not considered a chore as it may not have been something they were expected to do on a regular basis.

Recipes to Enjoy

Trash Hash Salad

2 cups cooked, broken spaghetti
2 cups shredded cabbage
1 large chopped green pepper
1 cup diced Monterey Jack cheese
1 small can garbanzo beans (chick-peas)
1 small onion, chopped
1/3 cup mayonnaise
1 tablespoon vinegar
1 teaspoon mustard
1 teaspoon sugar
1 teaspoon horseradish

Mix all ingredients in large bowl and toss. Enjoy with bread and a beverage. Serves 8-10.

Hoagies/Submarine Sandwiches

2 long loaves of French bread
Assorted sliced luncheon meat - e.g., ham, turkey, baloney, roast beef, pepperoni
Assorted sliced cheeses - e.g., American, Swiss, provolone
2 large sliced tomatoes
1 sliced onion
1 cup of lettuce, shredded
1 small bottle Italian salad dressing or mayonnaise

Slice the loaves of bread in half down the length of the bread. Open the bread and have participants layer meat and cheese to their liking. Top with shredded lettuce and tomato slices. Sprinkle with a dash of salad dressing for flavor. Close the loaf and cut into individual sandwich servings. Serves 6-8, depending on the length of the loaves of bread.

Make Your Own Ice Cream Sundaes

1 gallon vanilla ice cream
1 jar chocolate sauce
1 jar butterscotch/caramel topping
1 container whipped cream or "Cool Whip"
1 jar maraschino cherries
1 container chocolate or colored sprinkles
1 bag M&Ms
Fresh fruit, as desired
Nuts
Shredded coconut
Ground chocolate cookies

Use any or all of the above ingredients to create ice cream sundaes. Place each ingredient on a table in its own bowl with a serving spoon. Make sure all the ingredients are accessible to participants. Provide each individual with a bowl of vanilla ice cream. As they are able, participants can select their own toppings. This can be messy at times, but fun!

Surprise Chocolate Cake

1 package chocolate cake mix
1 16-ounce can well-drained and washed sauerkraut
Flat beer

Mix all ingredients listed on the cake mix package except for the liquid. Substitute flat beer for the exact amount of liquid required. Add the sauerkraut. Mix well. Use a large bowl for mixing so that participants can feel comfortable about not spilling ingredients. Bake as directed on package. This should be a very moist and delicious cake.

Kitchen Terms - Just for Fun

1. What does the term "baste" mean? Answer: To moisten food (usually meat) with juices from the pan or with other liquid

2. What is a scallion? Answer: An onion which has not developed a bulb

3. What is a soufflé? Answer: A dish made of milk and eggs; it is very airy and light, and tends to "puff up"

4. What is consommé? Answer: A clear broth that is highly seasoned

5. What does the term "puree" mean? Answer: To boil food to a pulp and put through a sieve

6. How do you knead bread? Answer: Place dough on a flat surface and work it by pressing down with the knuckles (or heel of your hand) and fold over several times

7. What is a demitasse? Answer: A half cup; usually a small after dinner cup of coffee

Men and Food

8. What does yeast do for bread dough? Answer: Makes the bread rise

9. What is the main ingredient in an omelet? Answer: Eggs

10. What part of an egg is the yolk? Answer: The yellow center (the outside is called the egg white)

11. What is the larger quantity, a teaspoon or a tablespoon? Answer: A tablespoon (three teaspoons equal one tablespoon)

12. What is lard? Answer: A soft fat rendered from pork, usually used for frying

13. Would you like the taste of baking chocolate? Answer: No; it is pure chocolate with no sugar, usually very bitter

14. What are you doing when you "broil" food? Answer: Cooking food at a very high temperature (400-500 degrees Fahrenheit), directly under radiant heat

15. How is food prepared if it is "sautéed"? Answer: The food is cooked gently in a small amount of fat or oil

Chapter 7

Sports

We couldn't discuss activity programming for men without mentioning sports in a big way. Baseball, football, boxing, wrestling, golf, and even the Olympics play a significant part in the lives of many men.

In the first half of the 20th century, America's favorite sport was baseball. Babe Ruth, Ty Cobb, Joe DiMaggio, Lou Gehrig, and Jackie Robinson were all heroes, admired by young and old alike. In fact, in 1927, Babe Ruth was considered the most popular man in the world! Memories of baseball may include thoughts of "Little League" or tossing the ball around with one's father. The men may recall attending a special big league game or participating in lighthearted family arguments over which team would win the big game. Some men take great pride in rattling off statistics on batting averages, football scores, seating capacities of stadiums, and team line-ups from years past.

Encourage discussion about whatever sports interest the men in your group. Memories of sporting events, whether as a participant or spectator, are very special.

Suggested Props

Baseball/glove/bat/cap
Football/helmet/t-shirt
Golf club/ball/tee
Tennis racket/ball
Basketball
Hot dogs
Baseball cards
Sports trophies
Sounds of a baseball game (see ElderSong Publications' "I Hear Memories")

Picture Sources

Time-Life Books - *This Fabulous Century, 1920-1930* and *1940-1950*

The First Fifty Years, Sugar Bowl Classics

The Lincoln Library of Sports, Volumes 1-20

The First 100 Years of Golf in America

The Yankees, Four Fabulous Eras of Baseball's Most Famous Team

(See Resource List for publishing information.)

Important Dates to Celebrate in Sports

January 1st: College football championship bowl games - the Rose Bowl, Cotton Bowl, Sugar Bowl, Orange Bowl, etc.

January 31st: Birthday of baseball player Jackie Robinson, born 1919. Elected to baseball hall of fame in 1962.

February 5th: Birthday of lifetime home run champ Hank Aaron, born 1934.

February 6th: Birthday of George Herman "Babe" Ruth, nicknamed the "Sultan of Swat," born 1895.

March 17th: Birthday of Bobby Jones, first golfer to win the Grand Slam, born 1902.

May: American Bicycle Month.

May 5th: Anniversary of baseball's first perfect game. In 1904, pitcher "Cy" Young did not allow a single player on the opposing team to reach first base.

May 6th: Birthday of baseball player Willie Mays, born 1931.

May 12th: Birthday of baseball player and coach Yogi Berra, born 1925.

May 24th: Anniversary of first baseball game played under the lights at Crosley Field in Cincinnati, 1934.

May 25th: Birthday of heavyweight boxing champion Gene Tunney, born 1898.

May 28th: Birthday of Olympian and football player Jim Thorpe, born 1888.

June: National Tennis Month.

June, second Monday: Beginning of National Little League Week, since 1959.

June 12th: Anniversary of National Baseball Hall of Fame; dedicated at Cooperstown, New York, in 1939.

June 16th: First squeeze play used in baseball in 1894 between the Yale and Princeton baseball teams.

June 24th: Birthday of heavyweight boxing champion Jack Dempsey, born 1895.

July 6th: Anniversary of first baseball all-star game in 1933 at Comiskey Park, Chicago. Babe Ruth hit a home run.

August 22nd: Anniversary of the International Yacht Race, now known as the America's Cup, first held in 1851.

September 12th: Birthday of Olympic runner Jesse Owens, born 1913.

September 22nd: Long Count Day, referring to the championship boxing match between Jack Dempsey and Gene Tunney in 1927.

September 24th: Anniversary of Babe Ruth's farewell to the Yankees in 1934.

September 25th: Anniversary of the first doubleheader in major league baseball in 1882.

October 20th: Birthday of baseball player Mickey Mantle, born 1931.

November 23rd: Anniversary of the first play-by-play broadcast of a football game in 1919.

November 25th: Birthday of baseball player Joe DiMaggio, born 1914.

December 18th: Birthday of baseball player Ty Cobb, born 1886.

Remember when...

..."Sunny" Jim Bottemley of the St. Louis Cardinals drove in 12 runs in a single game in 1924?

...Jack Dempsey faced heavyweight champion Gene Tunney at Chicago's Soldier's Field in 1927? There was great controversy over the length of the count after Tunney was downed by Dempsey's punch. By best estimates, the count was actually 14 seconds, giving Tunney extra time to stand up and eventually win the fight.

...Ernie Nevers played in the 1925 Rose Bowl with two broken ankles?

...Tennis player Bill Tilden had a serve that sped across the net at 163 m.p.h.?

...On April 11, 1923, Yankee Stadium opened as the nation's largest ball park, seating 65,000 fans? Babe Ruth celebrated opening day by hitting a home run. This stadium has been called "The House that Ruth Built."

...Jesse Owens broke three world track records in one afternoon, May 25, 1935?

..."Man O'War" set five American horse racing records in 1920?

...The Chicago Bears beat the Washington Redskins in 1940 by an astounding 73-0?

...Don Budge won the Grand Slam in tennis in 1938?

...Lou Gehrig became the first major league baseball player to hit four straight home runs in a single game on June 12, 1932?

...Football coach Knute Rockne led Notre Dame to 105 victories between 1919 and 1931?

...Boxer Sugar Ray Robinson turned pro in 1940 and won his next 40 bouts?

...Bill Terry hit over .400 in the 1930 baseball season?

...Duke's 1938 football team was undefeated, untied, and unscored upon when they lost the Rose Bowl game to Southern California?

...Satchel Paige pitched for the Kansas City A's when he was 59 years old on September 25, 1959?

Sports Trivia

1. What position did "Dizzy" Dean play for the St. Louis Cardinals? Answer: Pitcher

2. In boxing, who was the "Manassa Mauler"? Answer: Jack Dempsey

3. What did Jack Dempsey mean when he referred to his "Iron Mike"? Answer: His powerful right hand

4. Name the golfer who was the first to win the Grand Slam (four major golf tournaments) in 1930. Answer: Bobby Jones

5. Second baseman Jackie Robinson was the first African American to sign with the major leagues. What was his team? Answer: Brooklyn Dodgers

6. In the 1940s, what was Rocky Graziano's sport? Answer: Middleweight boxing

7. Hank Luisetti revolutionized what game with one-handed shots? Answer: Basketball

Sports

8. In 1937, "War Admiral" won the Triple Crown in what sport? Answer: Horse racing

9. What were Max Carey and Lou Brock famous for stealing in the 1920s? Answer: Bases, in major league baseball

10. Sportswriter Grantland Rice wrote, "Outlined against a blue-gray October sky, the four horsemen rode again." What football team was he referring to? Answer: Notre Dame

11. Who was the "Galloping Ghost" of Illinois? Answer: Red Grange (He left college football in 1925 to play with the Chicago Bears.)

12. According to golfer Bobby Jones, what was his "Calamity Jane"? Answer: His putter

13. In the 1940s, who was baseball's "Yankee Clipper"? Answer: Joe DiMaggio (He was the American League home run champion in 1937.)

14. For what major league baseball team did Satchel Paige play in the 1940s? Answer: The Cleveland Indians (He was a great pitcher and hitter.)

15. With what sport would you associate Barney Ross? Answer: Boxing (He was the 1933 welterweight boxing champion.)

16. What major league baseball team's batting line-up was known as "murderers' row" in 1927? Answer: The New York Yankees

17. Who was Bobby Feller? Answer: The first major league pitcher to hurl a no-hit, no-run game on opening day (Feller pitched this game in 1940 for the Cleveland Indians against the White Sox.)

18. Who was "Mr. Inside" on the Army football team, a fullback who won the Heisman Trophy in 1945? Answer: Doc Blanchard

19. In the 1920s, Ernie Nevers set a National Football League record by scoring 40 points in one game. He also played professionally in one other sport. Can you name the sport? Answer: Major league baseball

20. In professional golf, who was "Slammin' Sammy"? Answer: Sam Snead

21. What big mistake did Roy Riegels make in the 1925 Rose Bowl game? Answer: He ran 65 yards the wrong way with a fumble

22. Pancho Gonzales was known for his powerful serve in what sport? Answer: Tennis

23. In 1946, Marion Motley was the first African American to enter what major league sport? Answer: Football (He was a half-back for the Cleveland Browns.)

24. At one time, St. Louis had two major league baseball teams. Can you name them? Answer: The Cardinals and the Browns (The Browns later became the Baltimore Orioles.)

25. Why was the Notre Dame football team referred to as the "Nomads"? Answer: Because they played so many games on the road, even cross-country (Most college football teams of the time only played within their own region of the country.)

26. What was Ellsworth Vine's sport? Answer: Tennis (He was one of the few players who beat Bill Tilden.)

27. Were the Olympics held during World War II? Answer: No (The Olympics were held only once, in 1948, during the entire decade of the 1940s.)

28. What baseball player was known as the "Georgia Peach"? Answer: Ty Cobb

29. What sport involving a ball has the largest playing field? Answer: Polo (The field is 12.4 acres.)

30. Who was known as the "Home Run King" with 60 home runs in 1927? Answer: Babe Ruth

31. Who was Casey Stengel? Answer: Manager of the New York Yankees (Stengel led the team to five consecutive World Series titles between 1949 and 1953.)

32. In the 1941 World Series, catcher Mickey Owen nearly ruined his baseball career when he dropped the ball after the third strike in the last out of the ninth inning. What two major league baseball teams were playing in this game? (Hint: They were both from New York.) Answer: The New York Yankees and the Brooklyn Dodgers

33. What basketball player is known for scoring 100 points in a single game? Answer: Wilt Chamberlain

34. With what sport is Tom Harmon associated? Answer: College football (He played for Michigan.)

35. In 1941, a major league baseball team, the Boston Bees, changed its name to what? Answer: The Boston Braves

36. Name the two major league baseball teams that moved from New York to California. Answer: The New York Giants became the San Francisco Giants; the Brooklyn Dodgers became the Los Angeles Dodgers.

Questions for Discussion

1. What is your favorite sport? Did you participate in this sport as a child? Were you able to listen to this sport on the radio? Who was your favorite team?

2. Did you enjoy sports with your father? Did you ever have a memorable coach? Who taught you to throw a ball, swing a bat, or drive a golf ball?

3. Did you actively participate in any sport in high school or college? Did you win any trophies? Describe your memories of these school games.

4. Did you ever attend any major league games? Where? Is there a special game you recall? Did you ever see any of the famous sports heroes play? Who did you see? How did you feel?

5. Who is your favorite sports hero? Why? Did you ever collect player's autographs? Which autographs were you able to obtain?

6. Some professional players today receive contracts of several million dollars. How do you feel about that? Does a professional athlete have an obligation to set an example to the young people of today by maintaining a "clean" life-style? What did you think of Babe Ruth's antics? How do you feel about some of the life-styles of athletes today?

Sports

Active Sporting Ideas

1. Show a movie on sports, such as these:

   "The Natural"
   "Field of Dreams"
   "Rocky"
   "Dempsey"
   "The Babe Ruth Story"
   "Chariots of Fire" (set in 1924)
   "Golden Boy"
   "The Jessie Owens Story" (set in 1936)
   "The Lou Gehrig Story"
   "The Boys of Summer, the Brooklyn Dodgers"
   "Requiem for a Heavyweight"

   Serve hot dogs and coke.

2. Take the group to a local little league baseball game or a high school football game.

3. Have the men get together for a game of catch with a nearby children's group. Since you are involving children, you have the opportunity to use a softer ball and lighter equipment, thereby making the activity safer for everyone involved.

4. Take the men bowling. Many bowling establishments cheerfully accommodate handicapped individuals with assistive equipment.

5. Go miniature golfing. This is best done with a small group, no more than 8-10 men. Be sure to have several volunteers along to assist. Some areas have indoor courses and putting greens which are great for older adults who need to stay out of direct sunlight or heat. Indoor courses also mean you can plan in advance, even in unpredictable weather.

6. Play the Abbott and Costello "Who's on First" comedy sketch for the group (available from many libraries on cassette tape or video.) Mix in other comedy. Serve a snack. End the session by singing "Take Me Out to the Ball Game." (See page 33 for other sports songs.)

Chapter 8

Active Games

Physical activity is an essential part of life. Exercise not only keeps the body healthy but may also serve to alleviate depression, an all-too-frequent aspect of aging. Those who are cognitively impaired are often in fairly good physical condition. They need to exercise but may not have the opportunity to do so because of their need for constant supervision. Many men, in particular, have spent a lifetime being physically active. They may have played team sports as a hobby or participated with their children as a coach or scout leader.

Many individuals do not enjoy exercise just for the sake of movement. As activity coordinator, you need to be creative and make the exercise fun. On the whole, men enjoy games and friendly competition. Your biggest challenge is to make sure the games are adult in nature while remaining basic enough to keep from frustrating or intimidating the men. Walking around the block or to a local park when the weather cooperates should be a daily routine. This allows the men to interact with the out-of-doors, to experience the weather, and to connect with time of year. It also establishes a structure, something the men can count on and feel secure about each time they gather together. Outings, even if they aren't sports or game related, provide a wonderful source of enjoyable exercise. Exercise is good for the mind as well as the physical body.

Activities to Encourage Physical Exercise

Start a Walking Program

Set up a lap area around your parking lot, yard, or even within the facility. Measure this area so that you have a general idea of the distance, i.e., 1/4th or 1/8th of a mile. Encourage the men to walk (or wheel) around the area as many times as they can do it comfortably.

Make a large chart with each man's name on it and hang it somewhere visible in the meeting room. Help the men to chart their laps. Reward the men if they increase the number of laps or if they finish a goal of a certain number of laps over a period of time. By measuring the area and keeping track of laps, you can announce to the men how far they have traveled in a month or a year. Mark on a map the distance to a nearby city or resort area. Have a party when the men have hiked the distance to that location.

To really add purpose to the walking, ask friends and family members to pledge a penny (or a dollar) per lap. Give the funds raised to a favorite charity.

Go Fishing

This is easiest if you take the group to a pond where a license is not required and equipment is provided. Make sure there is a place for everyone to sit and that shade is available. Once you have caught the fish, have a fish fry back at the facility and give everyone a taste. Then sit around and tell big "fish" stories!

Hold a Senior Olympics

This takes a lot of planning and practice but can also be very worthwhile. Mark off certain areas of your yard or parking lot for the activity. Purchase ribbons or trophies for the winners. Be sure to have enough events so that everyone has an opportunity to participate and win an award. Your events can include:

a. **A frisbee toss** (discus throw). Award the blue ribbon to the one who tosses the frisbee the farthest.

b. **A short-distance walking race.** This means that heels must touch the ground with each step or the racer is disqualified for actually running. This race can be varied by changing the distance or by creating a relay. For a relay race, have the men positioned in various spots around the "track." The first racer carries a stick or beanbag which he hands to the next racer on the "track." He, in turn, hands the object to the racer further down the "track." This type of race is more complicated and is recommended for higher functioning individuals.

c. **A wheelchair race.** Staff members can push participants around the "track" in wheelchairs. This is a lot of fun and does not put a lot of physical stress on the participants.

d. **A golfing event.** Use a standard putter, golf ball, and a grassy outdoor area. If it is possible, you can actually dig a hole in the ground and stick a flag in it. Or use one of the plastic putting greens available in various activity catalogs. Award ribbons to those who can successfully drive the ball into the hole.

e. **A balloon volleyball game.** Divide the group into teams representing different countries participating in the Olympics. Set up a net and use a large balloon for the volleyball. This game can be played sitting down for those with physical disabilities. Keep score as you would in a regular volleyball game. May the best country win!

Challenge the Men to a Dart Game

There are many different types of "safe" dart games available through activity catalogs and educational supply stores. Often these darts will have rubber tips with no sharp edges. Select a dartboard that is adult in nature and whose darts are solid. If the darts are too lightweight, the men will have difficulty throwing them and become frustrated.

Play Croquet

If there is any yard area around your facility, a croquet game can be set up. Use colorful ribbon or flags to mark the wickets, which are nearly invisible to those with limited vision.

Play Horseshoes

This has been a popular game for many men. It is easy to set up outdoors and there are many varieties that can be used indoors. Select a set that appears adult, rather than a plastic set with childish colors. Our men's group has a park nearby with horseshoe pits already installed. In good weather, we take a weekly walk to the park, horseshoes in hand.

Play a Game of Bocce Ball

This is an Italian game of bowling played on a well-mowed lawn. The balls are smaller, lighter, and easier to handle. The game uses several brightly-colored balls that the players must roll across the lawn in order to land closest to the original ball. The game is easy to learn and fun to play.

Form a Hiking Club

At one time, several men in my group had been scout leaders and had thoroughly enjoyed hiking long distances in their younger years. Many areas around the country have well-kept hiking paths through parks or along rivers where the men can stroll or be pushed in wheelchairs. Look for paths that are level and, if possible, paved. For the men, these outings are different from the daily "walks." They are "hikes," where the men can experience nature and feel young once again.

Take the Men Dancing

Most likely, the men would be opposed to dancing with each other. (One of the men in our group has suggested that they each dance with a broomstick, but we think that's going a bit too far.) The men all agree that they love dancing with women. Contact local women's groups or dance instructors. Ask if they would be interested in presenting a dance program or dancing with the men. This does not have to be ballroom dancing.

Men often enjoy square dancing, line dancing, and watching belly dancing. In the event that women are not available, men do dance together in some countries around the world. I once played some Greek music for our men's group and found they all liked holding hands high in the air, clicking their fingers, and moving in a circle to the rhythm of the music. Many Russian, Israeli, and Irish dances also feature only men.

Play a Modified Game of Basketball

Use a beach ball or other lightweight ball and a low basket. The men can play standing or sitting in a chair. Score two points for each ball tossed into the basket. This can be for a single game or an ongoing championship.

Chapter 9

Women Men Have Loved

There's no doubt that men are fascinated with women. Our men's group can spend hours discussing cars, sports, and World War II, but inevitably the conversation leads to women. On some occasions, the men discuss wives and former girlfriends. On other days they dream of pin-up girls and sultry movie stars. It is on these occasions that I am absolutely convinced that men need time with just men. The group often engages in conversation that I doubt would occur if wives or other women were nearby.

During one gathering, the men were in a particularly giddy mood. One man began relating, in hilarious detail, how he persuaded a young college girl to kiss him. The other men enthusiastically joined in, telling stories of their first kisses. One group member had been slapped at a summer camp by a young lady who did not appreciate his somewhat awkward advances. Others described their fear when relating at a young age to those of the opposite sex. All agreed that they couldn't always understand female behavior. The men had discovered such a bond between them! The discussion ended with one man (who loves trains) remarking, "There's only one thing I've ever experienced that beats kissing a woman—the day I got to drive a trolley down Main Street!"

Name That Woman

Below are listed some of the women popular for their sex appeal during the first half of the twentieth century. Read the descriptions and see if the group can recall the woman's name. It is always best to use pictures with the descriptions to help encourage memories. (Picture sources: Eldergames' Flashback series; *This Fabulous Century*; Dover Publications' *Hollywood Glamour Portraits* or *Muray's Celebrity Portraits of the Twenties and Thirties*.)

Ask the men what they liked most about these women. Who were their favorites? Why? Do they recall seeing these women in the movies? If the group is unable to correctly guess names, use the list to encourage memories. Name the famous woman and see if the group can describe her. Provide the clues given and encourage discussion. Again, pictures are especially helpful with more impaired individuals.

1. Pin-up girl during World War II (usually wearing a bathing suit) - famous legs - blonde - married Harry James. Answer: Betty Grable

2. Sexy - sultry - blonde - buxom - "Come up and see me sometime." Answer: Mae West

3. Bubbly good looks - dance partner with Fred Astaire - charming - "The Gay Divorcee." Answer: Ginger Rogers

4. Beautiful - tough - witty - starred in screwball comedies - wisecracking blonde - married Clark Gable - killed in plane crash delivering war bonds. Answer: Carole Lombard

5. Voted Queen of Hollywood in 1937 - brunette - starred in "The Thin Man" - exotic femme fatale - green, almond-shaped eyes. Answer: Myrna Loy

6. Sexy - German - blonde - sang with the USO during WW II - great legs - starred in "Destry Rides Again" - sang "Lili Marlene." Answer: Marlene Dietrich

7. Vibrant brunette - sexy - beautiful - married Frank Sinatra and Mickey Rooney - appeared in "The Hucksters" and "Wanted." Answer: Ava Gardner

8. Strikingly beautiful - child actress - "National Velvet" - dark hair and violet eyes - married Richard Burton twice. Answer: Elizabeth Taylor

9. Blonde bombshell - "Red Dust" and "Dinner at Eight" - wise-cracking - slinky. Answer: Jean Harlow

10. Scarlet O'Hara in "Gone With the Wind" - was Blanche Dubois in "A Streetcar Named Desire" - green eyes. Answer: Vivien Leigh

11. Famous jazz and blues singer - "Lady Day" - sang with Artie Shaw Orchestra - wore a gardenia in her hair when she performed. Answer: Billie Holiday

12. Cool - courageous - tough - won Oscar for "Mildred Pierce" - dark hair and eyes - shoulder pads - "Mommie Dearest." Answer: Joan Crawford

13. "America's Sweetheart" - silent films - "Poor Little Rich Girl" - "Girl with the Curl" - married Douglas Fairbanks. Answer: Mary Pickford

14. Independent - strong-minded - paired with Spencer Tracy in nine films - "The Philadelphia Story." Answer: Katharine Hepburn

15. Strong personality - sharp tongue - "Jezebel" - "Of Human Bondage" - famous eyes. Answer: Bette Davis

16. Paris-born - throaty laugh - short bangs - won Oscar for "It Happened One Night." Answer: Claudette Colbert

17. Swedish - silent movies and talkies - "I vant to be alone" - "Anna Christie." Answer: Greta Garbo

18. Played Ilsa Lund in "Casablanca" - Swedish-born - "Joan of Arc." Answer: Ingrid Bergman

19. "The Sarong Girl" - south sea beauty image - road pictures with Hope and Crosby. Answer: Dorothy Lamour

20. Flapper - the "It" girl - earthy sensuality - flirtatious - red hair - boyish figure. Answer: Clara Bow

21. Played Dorothy in "Wizard of Oz" - singer/actress - "Over the Rainbow" - "Meet Me in St. Louis" - "Easter Parade." Answer: Judy Garland

22. "Norwegian Doll" - Olympic figure skater - actress. Answer: Sonja Henie

Related Activities

1. Show a movie featuring one of the many female movie stars of the past. "Woman of the Year," "Dinner at Eight," or "Casablanca" are a few good choices. Serve popcorn.

2. Invite a jazz dancer, ballet dancer, or even belly dancer to come in and entertain the men. Some areas have special arts performers who entertain senior groups. Contact a local theater group or choral group for leads.

3. Ask the men to bring in their wedding pictures to show to the group. Discuss wedding memories. Put together a photo display of the pictures. See if other group members and staff can recognize the men.

4. Invite spouses and women from the facility to join the men for a social hour. This can include festive food and ballroom dance music. Encourage dancing and movement to music.

5. Display pictures of popular women of today. Ask questions like these: Why are these women famous? How does their appeal differ from women of the past? What do you think of the assertive modern woman? How do you feel about "women's liberation"?

6. Invite teenagers from a school or youth group to visit the men. Discuss how women's roles have changed over the years. Do the men feel comfortable with these changes? Have the changes been beneficial to society as a whole?

7. Sing love songs. The men may enjoy singing "Let Me Call You Sweetheart," "You Are My Sunshine," and "Goodnight Sweetheart," just to name a few. Ask the men if there was a special song they sang to a loved one.

Questions for Discussion

1. Do you remember your first love? How old were you? Did you kiss her?

2. Where was your favorite spot for romance? The front porch swing? The rumble seat? On a moonlight stroll?

3. Describe a typical date in years past. How important was an automobile when dating? Where did you take the young lady? How expensive were the outings?

4. How did you meet your wife? Was it love at first sight? How did you know you were in love?

5. Describe how you proposed to your wife. Did you get down on your knees? Did you rehearse the proposal ahead of time? Did anyone help you?

6. Describe your wedding day. Were you nervous? Were you married in a church? Where did you go on your honeymoon?

7. Did you ever have a "crush" on an older woman, such as a teacher or a neighbor? Describe your feelings. Did you ever act on these feelings?

8. How important is appearance? Must a woman be attractive for you to be interested? How has your perspective on this changed over the years? How important is intelligence or sense of humor? What qualities do you look for in a woman?

9. If you were in the military, did you collect pin-up pictures of women? Where did you hang these pictures? Did you ever store one in your helmet? Do you recall your favorite pictures, perhaps Rita Hayworth or Betty Grable?

One Last Thought

Don't Forget Father's Day!

Annually, on the 3rd Sunday in June, Father's Day is a most appropriate time to honor the men in your facility. If they do not have children of their own, ask them if they would like to be honorary fathers for the day. This very important holiday was first suggested in 1910 by Mrs. John Dodd of Spokane, Washington. Later, President Calvin Coolidge recognized the day but it did not receive an official presidential proclamation until 1966.

In honor of Father's Day, provide carnations for the men to wear on their lapels. Feature pictures of the men throughout the facility with captions outlining their lifetime accomplishments. If the weather is warm, have an outdoor barbecue. Serve hamburgers, hot dogs, baked beans, and potato salad. Top it off with a chocolate cake. Later in the day, feature a video just for the men. (See sports movie ideas on page 41.)

Discuss the joys (and pitfalls) of fatherhood. Ask questions like these: Who are more difficult to raise, boys or girls? If you were never a father, was there a child who was important to you? What was your greatest joy as a father? How has fathering changed over the years? Have the changes been good ones? What special memories do you have of your own father?

Don't Forget Father's Day!

Resource List

Activity Resources

Bi-Folkal Productions. 809 Williamson Street, Madison, Wisconsin 53703. (608) 251-2818. High quality products including slides, old photos, and written material primarily for reminiscing. Many subjects geared for men.

Eldergames. 11710 Hunter Lane, Rockville, Maryland 20852. (800) 637-2604. Several photo sets of reminiscing products for seniors. Includes photos of automobiles, men's clothing, radio, travel, and famous personalities. Several trivia books are also available.

Polkarobics. 6 Oak Ridge, North Caldwell, New Jersey 07006. (201) 228-2006. A large variety of music and movement products, plus an entire section on train videos and several cassette tapes of old radio shows.

Potentials Development. 775 Main Street, Buffalo, New York 14203. (716) 842-2658. Activity ideas for reminiscing, exercising, crafts, and trivia.

Medical and Activities Sales. P.O. Box 4068, Omaha, Nebraska 68104. (800) 541-1898. Large variety of activity products from books to crafts to reminiscing material. Offers a horse racing game, as well as horseshoes and a shuffleboard set.

Geriatric Resources. 931 S. Semoran Blvd., Suite 200, Winter Park, FL 32792. (407) 678-1616. Hands-on materials for the Alzheimer's patient. Also offers videos and musical cassettes.

Pickett Enterprises. P.O. Box 11000, Prescott, Arizona 86304. (602) 778-1896. Carries a variety of programming material for activity coordinators.

Giant Photo. Box 406, Rockford, Illinois 61105. Offers inexpensive posters that are excellent resources for reminiscing.

Sources for Photographs

This Fabulous Century. Time Life Books, 1969-70. These books are now out of print, but are available in most local libraries. The volumes are divided by decade and are indispensable when conducting reminiscing programs with seniors. For men, the volumes contain photos of sports stars, labor leaders, and political figures, as well as automobiles and planes from the first seven decades of the twentieth century.

Dover Publications. 180 Varick Street, New York, New York 10014. They carry a variety of photograph books that feature famous personalities of the twentieth century.

***Ideals* magazine.** Ideals Publishing Corporation, P.O. Box 148000, Nashville, Tennessee 37214-8000. These magazines are full of nostalgic photographs, poetry, and short stories. They can be ordered by subscription (8 issues per year) or found in a local bookstore.

***Reminsce* magazine.** Reiman Publications, 5927 Memory Lane, P.O. Box 572, Milwaukee Wisconsin 53201-0572. A professionally-written magazine with beautiful full-color photographs. Topics include everyday life and memorable events from the first half of the 20th century.

***Good Old Days* magazine.** P.O. Box 337, Seabrook, New Hampshire 03874-0337. Offers nostalgic stories, poetry, and pictures. Often features copies of advertisements for men's clothing and accessories from years ago. Can be ordered by subscription.

Norman Rockwell's World of Scouting. By William Hillcourt. Harry N. Abrams, Inc., Publishers, New York. Includes 250 Rockwell illustrations of boy scouting over the past several decades.

The First 50 Years, Sugar Bowl Classics. By Marty Muli, Oxmoor House, Birmingham. Features football photographs.

The Lincoln Library of Sports Champions, Volumes 1 - 20. Frontier Press Company, Columbus, Ohio.

The First 100 Years of Golf in America. By George Peper and the editors of Golf Magazine, Harry N. Abrams, Inc., Pub., 1988.

The Yankees—The Four Fabulous Eras of Baseball's Most Famous Team. By Dave Anderson, Murray Chass, Robert Creamer, and Harold Rosenthal. Random House, New York.

Railways of the Twentieth Century. By Geoffrey Allen, Norton Publishing, 1983.

Handbook Guide to Old Time Classic Cars, 1885-1940. By Juraj Porizak, Arco Publishing, New York, 1985.

An American Journey by Rail. By Timothy Jacobson, Norton Publishing, 1988.

The Look of Cars, Yesterday, Today, and Tomorrow. By Henry B. Lent, Dutton Publishing, 1966.

Cars of the 1940s. By the editors of *Consumer Guide*, Beekman House Publishing, 1979.

Other Resources

National Senior Sports Association. 317 Cameron Street, Alexandria, Virginia 22344.

American Dance Therapy Association. 2000 Century Plaza, Suite 230, Columbia, Maryland 21044.

National Center on Arts and Aging. National Council on Aging, West Wing 100, 600 Maryland Ave., SW, Washington, D.C. 20024.

Chase's Calendar of Events. Contemporary Books, Department C, 180 North Michigan Ave., Chicago, Illinois 60601. Contains listing of significant events, past and present, for each day of the year.

Other resources published by ElderSong Publications, Inc.

"Christmas with ElderSong"

Down Memory Lane

"Eldersong: The Music and Gerontology Newsletter"

Funny Bones Don't Get Arthritis: Humor for the Young at Heart

Hidden Treasures: Music and Memory Activities for People with Alzheimer's

Holiday Mind Joggers

Hooray for Hollywood: Trivia and Puzzles for Those Today Who Remember Yesterday

"I Hear Memories!"

The Lost Chord: Reaching the Person with Dementia Through the Power of Music

Make Your Point!

Mind Joggers, Volumes 1, 2, and 3

Mind Stretchers

Moments to Remember

Musings, Memories, and Make Believe

Party Possibilities

Portal: A Dual-language (Spanish/English) Activity Book for Senior Learners

Puzzlers, Volumes 1 and 2

Remembering: Recall and Reminiscence Exercises for Memory-Impaired Older Adults

Say It With Music: Music Games and Trivia

"Sing-Along with ElderSong," Volumes 1 and 2

Travel Unlimited

What Do You Know? Trivia Fun and Activities for Seniors

Yesterdays: A Collection of Short Stories, Nostalgic Photographs, and Related Programming Materials for Seniors

You Be the Judge

ElderSong Publications, Inc. • P.O. Box 74, Mt. Airy, Maryland 21771 • 1-800-397-0533